Mental Health Journal for Christians

Mental Health Journal

FOR CHRISTIANS

Faith-Based Prompts to Improve Your Mind, Body & Spirit

CATHLEEN BEARSE, LCSW

ROCKRIDGE PRESS

Interior and Cover Designer: Amanda Kirk
Art Producer: Alyssa Williams
Editor: Eun H. Jeong
Production Editor: Rachel Taenzler
Production Manager: Jose Olivera

All images used under license from Shutterstock.com. Author photo courtesy of Jessica Brown of JW Brown Photography.

Paperback ISBN: 978-1-63878-880-5
R0

This journal belongs to

_____

Contents

Introduction

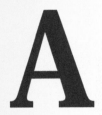s Christians, we have unlimited access to a God who loves us unconditionally and wants us to experience the fullness of His peace and joy, which He makes available to us at all times. And yet when we find ourselves in a difficult season or a time of prolonged uncertainty, it often feels difficult to access these gifts.

As a Christian myself and most recently as a foster mother, I, too, have struggled to access the peace and joy of God at times. It's definitely not easy to trust and find rest for my soul when my day-to-day life is filled with so much doubt and worry, especially where my children are concerned. From home visits and court dates to the daily stresses of parenting, it can feel pretty overwhelming at times. The antidote, I've found, is returning to God's truth, in addition to the practices I use and teach to my psychotherapy clients to overcome their own stress and anxiety.

Many people of Christian faith struggle to understand that they don't have to accept depression or anxiety or simply pray it goes away. Over the years, I have shared with clients the ways they can incorporate evidence-based therapeutic practices into their faith and vice versa. In fact, the most effective way to become (and stay) mentally healthy is to combine the two. Once we understand that faith and mental health aren't mutually exclusive, we can call upon both to more effectively reduce our stress, anxiety, and many other mental health concerns. I'm happy to show you how.

Each of the three sections in this book covers an important part of prioritizing your mental health. As you explore them, you'll discover how your feelings, thoughts, and relationships all play a role in keeping you mentally healthy.

My sincere hope in writing *Mental Health Journal for Christians* is to take the guesswork out of your mental health by providing a supportive and informative way to help busy Christians like you (and me!) avoid burnout, find focus, and live your best life. God has a lot to say about our mental health and well-being—He cares about it, and He wants us to care for it, too.

Lastly, please note that this journal is not meant to take the place of a meeting with a therapist, or diagnosing and treating a mental illness. If you are struggling with a mental illness or simply need additional support, please reach out to a local therapist (see page 156 for resources).

How to Use
This Journal

Many people are surprised to discover everything that a well-rounded mental health practice can encompass. Self-care is so much more than manicures and bubble baths; in fact, there is a myriad of options for healthy coping. Prayer and Bible reading are important self-care practices for people of Christian faith, but so are practices like setting healthy boundaries, getting proper rest, and engaging in a regular stillness practice such as meditation.

This journal was created to support you in both your faith and your quest for improved mental health. Since life is busy, full of responsibilities and demands on our time, each prompt is short—a verse from scripture that can encourage you, along with a question or two to get you thinking about what God has to say about your feelings, thoughts, and relationships.

The journal's three sections each cover an important aspect of your mental health—emotional well-being, psychological well-being, and social well-being—with the hopes of prompting reflection and shifting your perspective.

The prompts in this journal are intended to combine therapeutic practices with God's Word to help you recognize and reflect on what God has to say about your mental health. At the end of each section, you'll find a closing prayer as well as a related mental health practice that you can incorporate into your self-care routine.

Feel free to work through the journal from start to finish or complete the prompts in whatever order you feel will serve you most.

My prayer for you is that this journal will bless you as you prioritize your mental health and grow deeper in your faith. May it also be a reminder that God loves you and that the peace and joy He offers are available to you each and every day.

PART I

In Your Heart

WHEN WE EXPERIENCE STRONG EMOTIONS, WE ARE DOING MORE than mindfully observing the truth about what is happening in our lives. We tend to add to the truth, telling ourselves stories that include emotions like guilt or shame. The scriptures presented in this section of the book will help remind you of what God has to say about your feelings and about your emotional well-being.

Our feelings are *powerful*. When we have an emotion, we often feel it physically as well as emotionally. Our bodies have a physiological reaction to stress, anxiety, sadness, and anger. That reaction can make the feeling more difficult to handle. However, with practice, as some of the prompts in this section will guide you through, it's possible to notice when uncomfortable feelings arise (perhaps when you sense your body is beginning to react) and say to yourself, "Feelings are not facts," or "Just because I feel this doesn't mean it's true."

Additionally, the prompts in this journal will help you increase your resilience and capacity to be with your difficult emotions, rather than trying to change them or get rid of them. When we are willing to sit with our emotions, whether they feel pleasant or unpleasant, we allow room for God to guide us to the right course of action in dealing with them.

Unconditional Love

You have searched me, Lord, and You know
me. You know when I sit and when
I rise; You perceive my thoughts from afar.

PSALM 139:1-2

God knows you intimately, and when He looks at you, He is pleased
with what He sees, whether or not you *feel* like He is.

How does it make you feel to know that you are known so completely and loved so unconditionally? How can you rest in that
love today?

_____

_____

_____

_____

_____

_____

Grace

Therefore, there is now no condemnation
for those who are in Christ Jesus,
because through Christ Jesus the law
of the Spirit who gives life has set
you free from the law of sin and death.

ROMANS 8:1–2

When we fully receive the grace God offers us when we mess up, we are able to receive full freedom as well. Try to remember how God really thinks of you: as His own beloved child.

Write a letter to yourself, from God's perspective, about a mistake you are struggling to forgive yourself for.

Rest

The Lord replied, "My Presence will
go with you, and I will give you rest."

EXODUS 33:14

The pressure to succeed, to achieve, to be too busy for rest or connection tends to creep into our lives quietly. Eventually, it becomes
the status quo. God, however, wants to give us rest, both physical
and mental.

What are some ways you can enter into rest today that truly
refresh your mind and body? Consider the types of self-care that
have really rejuvenated you in the past. Next, choose at least one to
put into practice.

Gratitude

Every good and perfect gift is from above,
coming down from the Father of heavenly lights,
who does not change like shifting shadows.

JAMES 1:17

Practicing gratitude is a conscious choice. There will always be things going wrong in our lives, but there will also always be things going right. Counting our blessings has the power to change both our attitude and our life.

Use the following space to reflect on all the good and wonderful gifts in your life.

Self-Care

Don't you know that you yourselves
are God's temple and that
God's Spirit dwells in your midst?

1 CORINTHIANS 3:16

Practicing regular self-care is like preventive medicine for your mind, body, and soul. It helps you feel more peaceful and better equips you to regulate your emotions.

Caring for yourself is caring for God's temple. Can you think of anything you'd like to be doing that would benefit your mind, body, soul, or entire being?

Equanimity

I have told you these things, so that in me you
may have peace. In this world you will have trouble.
But take heart! I have overcome the world.

JOHN 16:33

If you are struggling to maintain peace in a stressful or chaotic time
of life, spend some time meditating on scriptures or quotes that
are meaningful to you. Read them often, speak them aloud, journal
about them. Retrain your brain to walk by faith and not by sight.

Write out some verses that bring peace to your heart.

Hope

Because You are my help,
I sing in the shadow of Your wings.

PSALM 63:7

Even when things appear hopeless, rest assured, that is not the case. We may get hurt or experience heartbreak–but our hope is real and the rescue will come. Hope allows us to sing and have joy even in the midst of pain.

Write about a time when things seemed hopeless but eventually worked out for you.

God's Promise

But in keeping with His promise we are
looking forward to a new heaven and
a new earth, where righteousness dwells.

2 PETER 3:13

As followers of Christ, we can be confident that our earthly experience is temporary, and we look forward to our heavenly home where everything will be filled with God's righteousness.

What difficult task or circumstance are you facing right now that feels overwhelming? How can the hope of heaven bring you comfort and the strength to find rest and positivity now?

The Future

Commit to the Lord whatever you do,
and He will establish your plans.

PROVERBS 16:3

The concept of nonattachment teaches us to live without rumination or fixation on what might happen or what we want and, instead, to fully accept life as it happens and experience it without expectation or judgment. The sooner we learn to entrust our plans to God, the more peace we will have.

Write a prayer to God committing your future plans to Him, knowing that He will establish them all according to His perfect will.

....

....

....

....

....

....

....

....

....

....

....

....

....

....

....

....

....

....

Freedom

_____

Now the Lord is the Spirit, and where
the Spirit of the Lord is, there is freedom.

2 CORINTHIANS 3:17

_____

Many people feel as though God wants to limit their freedom, when nothing could be further from the truth.

Are there ways you are feeling limited right now or situations in which you don't feel free? Consider some ways that you can act to give yourself more freedom in these areas and leave the rest in God's capable hands.

_____

_____

_____

_____

_____

Trust

Trust in the Lord with all your heart
and lean not on your own understanding.

PROVERBS 3:5

Many people mistakenly make faith about how they feel; the truth is, we can't always trust our feelings because they are constantly changing. But God never changes; He is always steadfast, always loving, always good.

How would your life look different if you were able to trust in the Lord with all your heart?

....

....

....

....

....

Desires

But if from there you seek the Lord your God,
you will find Him if you seek Him
with all your heart and with all your soul.

DEUTERONOMY 4:29

While there's nothing wrong with wanting to be happy or success-
ful, it's important not to make those our greatest desires in life. God
wants us to seek *Him* first because He truly knows what's best for us.

Make a list of things you are "seeking" in your life. Do you feel
they align with what God desires for you?

Thankfulness

So then, just as you received Christ Jesus as Lord,
continue to live your lives in Him, rooted and built
up in Him, strengthened in the faith as you
were taught, and overflowing with thankfulness.

COLOSSIANS 2:6–7

Thankfulness is a serious game changer for not only our faith but also our mental health. We always have the choice to be grateful or to complain. We can choose either contentment or discontentment in any given moment.

Use the space below to "overflow with thankfulness." Let your grateful thoughts about everything in your life, from personal to work to spiritual, flow from your heart onto the page.

Stillness

He says, "Be still, and know that I am
God; I will be exalted among the nations,
I will be exalted in the earth."

PSALM 46:10

Before you get going today, sit in stillness and quiet for 5 or
10 minutes. Mindfully take some deep breaths and notice what
thoughts arise. The more you practice stillness, the more you will
want to.

What emotions were you experiencing before and after you sat in
stillness? What changed for you after taking time to mindfully sit in
God's presence?

Belonging

And you also are among those Gentiles
who are called to belong to Jesus Christ.

ROMANS 1:6

To the people-pleasers, chronic perfectionists, and anyone who feels unworthy sometimes, *you belong.* Just you, flaws and all. You don't need to spend your precious life fighting to prove your worth. You are loved by God, dearly, unconditionally–that means without condition, without exception–and you belong to Him.

What does it mean to you personally that you belong to Jesus?

Grief

———————

... and provide for those who grieve in Zion—to
bestow on them a crown of beauty instead
of ashes, the oil of joy instead of mourning, and
a garment of praise instead of a spirit of despair.

ISAIAH 61:3A

———————

Let your pain be your teacher. In every painful circumstance, ask
yourself, "What was in my control? What was out of my control?"
You may not be able to control much, but you *can* control yourself
and your responses to people and life.

What can you praise God for even in the midst of pain or grief?

Strength

Finally, be strong in the
Lord and in His mighty power.

EPHESIANS 6:10

Failure doesn't equal defeat. We can make mistakes and learn from them, coming out stronger and more courageous on the other side. No matter what happened yesterday, learn from it, and most importantly, be gentle with yourself.

What does it mean to "be strong in the Lord"? What are some ways you can access His mighty power today?

Authenticity

I praise You because I am fearfully
and wonderfully made; Your works are
wonderful, I know that full well.

PSALM 139:14

Being our real, authentic selves is a gift to ourselves and our
loved ones. God made us unique for a purpose, and our life and
relationships improve when we allow our true selves to shine
through.

Write a prayer to God thanking Him for making you uniquely
you, and ask Him for release from feelings of condemnation or any
regrets you are struggling with.

Resilience

———————

I will refresh the weary and satisfy the faint.

JEREMIAH 31:25

———————

Often people wake up in the morning, and immediately their mind jumps to how little sleep they got, how tired they are, or how much they have to do that day. Instead, train yourself to remember what is going well and the source of your strength.

How can focusing on the positive strengthen you and make you more resilient? Jot down a few things you can remember for tomorrow morning.

....

....

....

....

....

....

Guidance

Guide me in Your truth and teach me,
for You are God my Savior,
and my hope is in You all day long.

PSALM 25:5

We must learn to stop looking around and comparing ourselves to others, especially people we only know on the internet and social media. We must keep our eyes fixed on God's truth, rather than what people think of us.

What does God's truth say about our value? What are some ways you can keep God's truth in your heart all day long?

God's Love

"Though the mountains be shaken and the hills
be removed, yet my unfailing love for you will not
be shaken nor my covenant of peace be removed,"
says the Lord, who has compassion on you.

ISAIAH 54:10

Whether you are celebrating a huge victory or putting the pieces back together after a crippling defeat, whether you have everything you could ever want or you are desperately wondering if there's more to life than this . . . *God loves you.*

Write down a failure you have experienced and a success you have experienced. How does your awareness of God's love and compassion for you move you to a greater sense of peace?

Joy

Though you have not seen Him, you love
Him; and even though you do not see Him
now, you believe in Him and are filled
with an inexpressible and glorious joy.

1 PETER 1:8

God offers joy to us that cannot be taken away, if we would only
receive it. What is the difference between happiness and joy? How
does deep faith relate to inexpressible joy?

List several reasons why believing in God has the capacity to
fill you with glorious joy. Then list some ways you've experienced
joy lately.

Coping

_____

Peace I leave with you; my peace I give to you.
I do not give to you as the world gives. Do not let
your hearts be troubled and do not be afraid.

JOHN 14:27

_____

If you feel yourself trapped in fear and anxiety over a what-if situation, go ahead and let it play out in your head to the worst possible end. Next picture what you would do, how you would cope, and who you would call on for help.

Describe a situation you have been anxious about and what you would do to cope.

_____

_____

_____

_____

_____

Self-Love

But who are you, a human being, to talk back
to God? "Shall what is formed say to the one who
formed it, 'Why did you make me like this?'"

ROMANS 9:20

Why love ourselves? Because we were made for love, and we cannot love well if we don't have a right view of ourselves. God made us exactly how we are in order to be exactly who we are, and He doesn't make mistakes.

Make a list of things you genuinely love about yourself.

Practice: Contemplative Prayer

Contemplative prayer is a practice we can come back to again and again when we want to tune in to our heart and the guidance of the Holy Spirit. In this type of prayer, we ask God a question, preferably aloud, and then we sit in stillness. Give yourself several minutes to sit and receive whatever wisdom you feel in your heart or hear directly from God.

It is most helpful to begin with a list of questions in mind before you start a contemplative prayer session, and have a journal and pen handy so you can jot down anything that you receive.

Here are a few examples of questions to get you started:

- What should I focus on for my spiritual health this week?

- How can I improve my physical health today?

- What key relationships should I focus on this week?

- What should I do about _____ [a current struggle you are having]?

This type of prayer helps us quiet the noise of the outer world and tune in to our heart, allowing space for God to speak directly to us. So many answers are available to us when we are willing to be still and listen.

Closing Prayer

Heavenly Father, thank You for the way that You care about my mental health. Thank You for wanting the absolute best for me.

I pray that You would show me how to be more like You; make my heart more like Yours. Help me grow closer to You and closer to the people in my life by putting into practice the things that I am learning from Your Word.

I pray that You would be with me as I seek to improve my mental health. Help me understand how to deal with anxiety, stress, and sadness as they arise. Help me glorify You in my heart and in my life. Allow others to see You in me each day. I pray that You would help me have continuous wisdom from You about how to cultivate peace and gratitude in my heart and in my life. Help me remember that Your peace and Your joy are always available to me.

Please protect my heart from anything that is not from You and help me keep Your truth stored in my heart each day. Thank You for loving me so perfectly.

In Jesus's name, amen.

PART II

In Your Thoughts

MANY OF US STRUGGLE WITH INTRUSIVE THOUGHTS LONG BEFORE we are ever aware of their presence. Automatic thoughts that take us out of the present moment can be particularly difficult to manage, but by bringing greater awareness to our experiences, moods, and thoughts, we can enable ourselves to process intrusive thoughts and take away a lot of their power.

Uncomfortable and intrusive thoughts have a greater chance of taking over if we don't understand how or why they are happening. When we understand the underlying triggers that take us out of the present moment, we are better equipped to cope effectively and reduce the chances of them recurring.

Most intrusive thoughts are considered to be some type of cognitive distortion—these are negative automatic thoughts that can make peace of mind seem nearly impossible if they go unchecked. Black-or-white thinking, catastrophizing, and jumping to conclusions are all examples of common cognitive distortions.

This section of the journal will guide you through scriptures and prompts to help you recognize and overcome these disruptive and destructive thought patterns. In His Word, God offers us encouragement and practical solutions for keeping our thoughts healthy, resulting in more peace and less stress and anxiety.

God's Presence

Blessed are those who have learned to acclaim
You, who walk in the light of Your presence, Lord.

PSALM 89:15

When we praise and acclaim God, we become more aware of God's presence and blessings in our lives.

What does it mean to walk in the light of God's presence? How do you think being reminded of God's presence continuously being with you can improve your mental health and thoughts?

Peace

. . . the Lord make His face shine on you
and be gracious to you; the Lord turn His
face toward you and give you peace.

NUMBERS 6:25-26

God desires for us to have peace, and He offers it to us freely
through our continuous connection with Him.

Write a prayer asking God to be gracious to you and give you
peace. Be specific about current worries, struggles, and feelings of
being overwhelmed, and don't censor yourself—pour your heart out
before the Lord.

Self-Talk

The Lord Your God is with you, the Mighty
Warrior who saves. He will take great delight
in you; in His love He will no longer rebuke
you, but will rejoice over you with singing.

ZEPHANIAH 3:17

For many of us, it's easier to focus on all the things we don't love
about ourselves than the things we do. Positive self-talk is something
we must work to cultivate.

Does knowing that God delights in you change the way you think
about yourself? Why or why not? Write down a few positive things
God would say about you.

Anxiety

———————

Cast all your anxiety on Him
because He cares for you.

1 PETER 5:7

———————

God invites us to "cast our anxiety" on Him. Can you take a moment
to visually picture yourself doing that?

Make a list of your current anxieties, and then picture yourself
literally casting them, or throwing them, into God's hands. Describe
how it feels to imagine this, and write down what comes to mind.

....

....

....

....

....

....

Work Ethic

Whatever you do, work at it with all your heart,
as working for the Lord, not for human masters.

COLOSSIANS 3:23

Sometimes we are fortunate to enjoy our work, and yet there are some tasks we must complete that seem to bring us no joy whatsoever.

List the jobs you currently find yourself in charge of that you do not enjoy. Brainstorm some ways you can bring more fun or enjoyment to these tasks.

Transforming Your Thoughts

The mind governed by the flesh
is death, but the mind governed by
the Spirit is life and peace.

ROMANS 8:6

As Christians, we have access to the Holy Spirit at all times.

What does the phrase "governed by the Spirit" mean to you? What are some practical ways you can ensure your mind is being governed by God's Spirit? What benefits do you think you'll experience as you allow this transformation of your thoughts to take place?

Control

A person's steps are directed by the Lord.
How then can anyone understand their own way?

PROVERBS 20:24

While it may be tempting to plan our lives from start to finish, the reality is that God is in control and we are not.

Write about a time you tried to control an outcome (or a person), only for it to cause you frustration. How can you leave room for God to have *His* way next time?

Morning Routine

In the morning, Lord, You hear my voice;
in the morning I lay my requests
before You and wait expectantly.

PSALM 5:3

While there's no rule stating that you must spend time with God first thing in the morning, there are numerous scriptures that point to the benefits of starting our day with an awareness of God's presence.

Create a morning routine for yourself that includes time with God in some way–through praying, reading scripture, or even using this journal.

Intrusive Thoughts

We demolish arguments and every
pretension that sets itself up against the
knowledge of God, and we take every
thought and make it obedient to Christ.

2 CORINTHIANS 10:5

Many of us go about our lives being swept away by our automatic thoughts rather than taking an active role in our thoughts.

What are some intrusive thoughts you have been having lately that you would like to make obedient to Christ by replacing with a truth from His Word?

Worries

There is no fear in love. But perfect love drives
out fear, because fear has to do with punishment.
The one who fears is not made perfect in love.

1 JOHN 4:18

God tells us that because we are loved perfectly by Him, we have
nothing to fear. God's love for us never changes, even if our feelings may.

Can you think of a time when feeling unloved or unappreciated
caused you to feel anxious or fearful? Write a list of times you have
felt worried lately, and remind yourself how perfectly loved you are.

....

....

....

....

....

Knowing God's Peace

———————

Grace and peace be yours in abundance through
the knowledge of God and of Jesus our Lord.

2 PETER 1:2

———————

Grace and peace are available to us *in abundance* through our knowledge of God and His Son Jesus when we seek it.

Make a list of ways you have gotten to know the people you are closest with. Now make a list of ways you can get to know God better so you can experience His abundance of peace.

Weariness

The Sovereign Lord has given me a well-instructed
tongue, to know the Word that sustains the
weary. He wakens me morning by morning, wakens
my ear to listen like one being instructed.

ISAIAH 50:4

When we are feeling weary, God wants us to turn to Him and rely on His never-ending strength. We can find many examples in scripture of God's desire for us to be sustained by Him.

Write out some of your favorite verses that remind you that God offers us His strength in our times of weariness.

....

....

....

....

....

Comfort

————————

Even though I walk through the darkest valley,
I will fear no evil, for You are with me;
Your rod and Your staff, they comfort me.

PSALM 23:4

————————

In difficult circumstances, we often turn to other people or things. Take a moment to consider who or what you typically turn to for comfort.

How do you think God's comfort could be more beneficial than your current comfort choices? What are some ways you can experience His comfort first, rather than turning to other people or things?

Feeling Overwhelmed

In the same way, the Spirit helps us
in our weakness. We do not know what we
ought to pray for, but the Spirit Himself
intercedes for us through wordless groans.

ROMANS 8:26

Can you think of a time when you felt so overwhelmed that you didn't even know what to pray for? God tells us His Holy Spirit intercedes for us in these times.

What feelings arise for you as you reflect on this? What are you currently feeling overwhelmed about that you can offer up to the Holy Spirit today?

Rejoicing

_____

The Lord has done it this very day;

let us rejoice today and be glad.

PSALM 118:24

_____

God tells us we can rejoice in _all_ circumstances. Joy is something we can choose, even when we don't necessarily feel happy.

Journal about some things God has done for you lately, and then write down some ways you can rejoice over them today. Choose at least one to put into practice.

....

....

....

....

....

....

Troubles

_____

Let us then approach God's throne of grace
with confidence, so that we may receive mercy
and find grace to help us in our time of need.

HEBREWS 4:16

_____

God tells us He wants us to approach Him with confidence in our time of need. One way to increase our confidence and strengthen our faith is by reflecting on past times that God has delivered us out of our troubles.

List as many past struggles as you can that God has already taken care of for you.

_____

_____

_____

_____

_____

Faith

———————

For we live by faith, not by sight.

2 CORINTHIANS 5:7

———————

God desires us to live by faith, or by trust in Him, not merely by what we see happening around us.

What difficult things do you see happening in the world lately that may be causing you to doubt God's goodness or power? Next to each one, write an affirmation of God's character despite what you see.

Fears

———————

I sought the Lord, and He answered me;
He delivered me from all my fears.

PSALM 34:4

———————

Try as we might to avoid them, fear and anxiety are natural parts of life. As uncomfortable as fear is, it benefits us if we allow it to make us more aware of our need for God.

Write a prayer to God asking Him to deliver you from everything you are currently feeling fearful or worried about.

———————————————————————————————
———————————————————————————————
———————————————————————————————
———————————————————————————————
———————————————————————————————
———————————————————————————————
———————————————————————————————

Abundance Mindset

Therefore do not worry about tomorrow,
for tomorrow will worry about itself.
Each day has enough trouble of its own.

MATTHEW 6:34

God is a God of abundance, though we have a natural human tendency to focus on the negative or scarcity most of the time.

Make a list of everything you see, big or small, that is a sign of God's infinite abundance and provision in your life. Let it remind you that today is a blessing and tomorrow is, too—no matter what it holds.

Frustration

"For my thoughts are not your thoughts,
neither are your ways my ways," declares the Lord.
"As the heavens are higher than the earth,
so are my ways higher than your ways and my
thoughts than your thoughts."

ISAIAH 55:8-9

While it might feel frustrating to not always understand "why" God allows certain things to happen to us, it benefits our mental health to trust that He is in control and His thoughts and ways are much different from ours.

Journal about some times when a stressful or trying circumstance actually worked out for your good in some way.

Perseverance

And let us run with perseverance
the race marked out for us.

HEBREWS 12:1B

We don't always get to choose our course; sometimes we are dealt a hand we would rather not play. But we can choose *how* we run our course; we can choose our attitude while we play that tricky hand.

Create a list of messages from God's Word that will encourage you to persevere through difficult times.

God's Provision

The lions may grow weak and
hungry, but those who seek the
Lord lack no good thing.

PSALM 34:10

One of the names of God found in scripture is Jehovah Jireh, which translates to "the Lord will provide."

Think back to the most abundant times in your life, and write down the ways you saw God provide for you. Even during a time when you had much less, how did God provide for your physical and spiritual needs?

God's Counseling

But very truly I tell you, it is for your good that I am going away. Unless I go away, the Advocate will not come to you; but if I go, I will send Him to you.

JOHN 16:7

Jesus refers to the Holy Spirit as an Advocate and, in other places in scripture, as a Counselor.

Imagine you are sitting in a counselor's office. What would you want to discuss with them right now? Write about it here, and when you're finished, read it aloud to the Holy Spirit, as if in conversation with Him.

Praise

Sing to the Lord, all the earth;

proclaim His salvation day after day.

Declare His glory among the nations,

His marvelous deeds among all peoples.

1 CHRONICLES 16:23-24

You don't have to be an amazing vocalist to sing praises to God, and doing so is an amazing way to practice gratitude and remind yourself of God's power.

Write a poem or song of praise to God in the space provided, and don't hold back. Unabashedly declare the marvelous deeds He has done in your life.

Practice: Cultivating Gratitude Every Day

It can be very difficult to turn our negative thoughts around when we're going through a difficult season in life or even just having a bad day. One of the best antidotes to negativity is a regular gratitude practice.

On even the worst days, there are blessings to count. By training your thoughts to look for the good, you will be more adept at doing so in the future.

For a fun twist on a gratitude practice, place a cup or jar in a designated spot for a month. Cut some blank paper into strips, and place the strips and a pen or pencil next to your jar. Each time you have a spare moment, grab a slip of paper and quickly jot down something you are grateful for. At the end of the month, you can read through all the papers in the jar.

If you live with others, feel free to invite them to join you in this exercise. Soon your cup will truly be running over with the blessings you and your loved ones have acknowledged throughout the month.

Closing Prayer

Heavenly Father, thank You so much that You desire healthy thoughts for me. Please help me keep my thoughts centered on You. I pray that You would guide me to Your truth about what it means to keep my thoughts healthy. Please guard my mind against thoughts that are not from You. Show me how to keep my thoughts focused on the things that are important to You.

Please keep my mind resilient and strong, and help me remember that I can take every thought and hold it up against the truth of Your Word. Please give me wisdom each day and help me be more like You. I pray that my thoughts would glorify You and that You would increase my peace each day. Help my thoughts lead me to live peacefully and joyfully.

I ask You to help me return to the present moment each time my thoughts wander away from it. Whenever I am triggered by a difficult person or situation, please help me be still and listen for Your wisdom for how to respond. Allow me to be more aware of Your presence with me each day.

In Jesus's name, amen.

PART III

In Your Community

OUR RELATIONSHIPS WITH FAMILY, FRIENDS, COLLEAGUES, AND THE larger community can greatly enrich our lives, and this is God's will—He desires for us to nourish and be nourished by the people around us. However, navigating relationships can be tricky sometimes, and even the people we love most can cross our boundaries and frustrate, annoy, or even hurt us from time to time. Thankfully, God has a lot to say about building and maintaining healthy relationships. From setting boundaries to navigating disagreements, the Bible provides guidance that will not only draw us closer to God but also the people we care about.

When we have a sound understanding of how God wants us to handle difficult people and situations, we can preserve and protect our mental health. When we look to God's Word for advice about issues like people-pleasing, dealing with unhealthy relationships, and understanding people who seem incredibly different from ourselves, we find an abundance of wisdom for these topics and many more.

This section of the journal will give you the opportunity to assess your current relationships as they pertain to your mental health *and* your faith.

People Changing

Jesus Christ is the same
yesterday and today and forever.

HEBREWS 13:8

Sometimes we forget that even the people we know best are always changing. At times, they might say or do something that surprises us or even hurts us. But Jesus never changes.

How can you take comfort in knowing that Jesus will remain constant in your life? How can you rest in this confidence when people you love disappoint you?

Complaining

Do everything without grumbling or arguing,
so that you may become blameless and pure,
"children of God without fault in a warped
and crooked generation." Then you will shine
among them like stars in the sky.

PHILIPPIANS 2:14–15

Complaining rarely makes us feel better, and it doesn't really solve our problems.

Write about the last thing you complained or vented about to someone. Spend some time journaling about why you felt the need to do so and whether you feel it truly improved your situation. Why or why not?

Resentment

_____

Do not fret because of those who are evil
or be envious of those who do wrong.

PSALM 37:1

_____

When we see people seemingly getting away with doing the wrong thing, it can be very disheartening. God tells us not to fret about what other people are doing and not to envy them.

Write about a few people who have caused you to feel jealous or resentful, then brainstorm some ideas to help you release these feelings today.

Honesty

Therefore, rid yourselves of all
malice and all deceit, hypocrisy, envy,
and slander of every kind.

1 PETER 2:1

Telling the truth and speaking kind words are ways that God desires for us to love one another. Doing so also improves our mental health by helping us live with integrity for what we believe.

Write about a situation in which you found it difficult to be completely honest or kind. How did you feel after this encounter?

The Most Important Relationship

By faith Abraham, when God tested him,
offered Isaac as a sacrifice. He who had embraced
the promises was about to sacrifice his one and
only son, even though God had said to him,
"It is through Isaac that your offspring will be
reckoned." Abraham reasoned that God could
even raise the dead, and so in a manner of
speaking he did receive Isaac back from death.

HEBREWS 11:17–19

Abraham was willing to part with his only son because he trusted
God and valued his relationship with Him more than anything else.

Who are the most important people in your life? Write a prayer
thanking God for the blessing of these loved ones, and ask Him to
help you keep Him first in your life.

Blessing Others

This is how you are to bless the Israelites.
Say to them: "The Lord bless you and
keep you; the Lord make His face shine
on you and be gracious to you . . . "

NUMBERS 6:23–25

One of the best ways we can improve our mental health is by caring for others.

Write about some words and actions that people have used to bless you in the past. How did their kindness toward you make you feel? List some ways you hope to bless others through words and deeds in the near future.

Taming the Tongue

Those who consider themselves religious
and yet do not keep a tight rein
on their tongues deceive themselves,
and their religion is worthless.

JAMES 1:26

We can consider what triggers us most often when it comes to speaking words we might later regret. Bringing awareness to these triggers can help us reduce their intensity in the future.

What does it mean to keep a tight rein on your tongue? In what ways do you currently struggle to do so? Reflect and write about this.

Living in Peace

Make every effort to live in peace
with everyone and to be holy; without
holiness no one will see the Lord.

HEBREWS 12:14

We all have people in our lives who are difficult to deal with. We can't change them, but we can change how we choose to deal with them.

Who are the people you find it most difficult to live in peace with? Why is it a challenge? Write about how you might strengthen your resolve to live in peace with them going forward. Choose one action step to take today.

Fellowship

Glorify the Lord with me;

let us exalt His name together.

PSALM 34:3

When we come together with other believers to praise God and share stories about what He is doing in our lives, it pleases Him and improves our well-being.

Journal about the wonderful things God has done in your life. Choose someone to share these stories with, and ask them what God is doing in their life right now.

Healthy Helping

Yet it was good of you
to share in my troubles.

PHILIPPIANS 4:14

Sharing in someone's troubles doesn't mean involving ourselves to an unhealthy degree such that it becomes a trouble for us; rather, God wants us to be an encouragement to those who are going through hard times.

Journal about a time when you got too involved with someone else's struggle. What would be a healthier way to respond?

Praying for Others

_____

For this reason, since the day we heard
about you, we have not stopped praying for you.
We continually ask God to fill you with
the knowledge of His will through all the wisdom
and understanding that the Spirit gives.

COLOSSIANS 1:9

_____

As Christians, we know that prayer is powerful; it is also one of the many ways God uses us in the lives of others.

Make a list of the people you want to be more intentional about praying for. You can ask them for their prayer requests, as well as anything God puts in your heart to ask for on their behalf.

Saying No

Be shepherds of God's flock that is under
your care, watching over them—not
because you must, but because you are
willing, as God wants you to be; not pursuing
dishonest gain, but eager to serve.

1 PETER 5:2

It's okay to say no to something when we can't give it without resentment.

Write about a time someone asked you to do something and you agreed only because you felt you *should*. Write out several ways to gently say no when someone asks you to do something that you can't joyfully give of yourself.

Slander

Though they plot evil against you and devise
wicked schemes, they cannot succeed.

PSALM 21:11

Have you ever felt like someone was out to get you? Whatever their
reasoning, it can cause you to feel helpless and hopeless, especially
if their plans to slander or harm you seem to be succeeding.

Journal about a time when you felt this way and how God may
have been using the situation for your good.

Unity

My prayer is not for them alone. I pray also
for those who will believe in me through
their message, that all of them may be one,
Father, just as You are in me and I am in You.

JOHN 17:20-21A

In a world that feels more divided than ever, we must remember
that God desires unity for His children.

What are some ways you have seen divisiveness in your relationships or surroundings lately? What feelings arise for you as you bring
awareness to this lack of unity? What is one thing you can do today
to foster unity?

Loneliness

A father to the fatherless, a defender
of widows, is God in His holy dwelling.
God sets the lonely in families, He leads
out the prisoners with singing.

PSALM 68:5-6A

Oftentimes when we feel lonely, we may think there is nothing we can do to change our situation. In reality, there are many ways we can combat loneliness and connect with others.

What are your favorite ways to connect with others? Use the space provided to plan activities you can do whenever you feel sad or alone.

Releasing Negativity

If you do away with the yoke of oppression,
with the pointing finger and malicious talk,
and if you spend yourselves in behalf of the
hungry and satisfy the needs of the oppressed,
then your light will rise in the darkness, and your
night will become like the noonday.

ISAIAH 58:9–10

Whether someone speaks maliciously about us or we speak poorly of someone else, the negative effects on our mood are the same. These emotions will stay with us for as long as we give them energy.

Write a prayer to God asking Him to help you release feelings of malice toward anyone who has hurt you.

Connection

Every day they continued to meet
together in the temple courts.
They broke bread in their homes and ate
together with glad and sincere hearts.

ACTS 2:46

Healthy relationships develop over time when we prioritize sharing life with others and having fun together.

Reflect on some memorable moments you have spent sharing life with others. How can you ensure that connection with your loved ones remains a priority despite the busyness of life? How do you think this will improve your mental health? Write your thoughts.

Advocacy

Religion that God our Father accepts
as pure and faultless is this: to look after orphans
and widows in their distress and to keep oneself
from being polluted by the world.

JAMES 1:27

God tells us that the poor will always be with us but that He wants us to care for them in their distress.

Make a list of marginalized or vulnerable populations that you have a heart for. What are some ways you can advocate for them? How can you use your time and resources to help reduce their suffering?

....

....

....

....

Forgiveness

Bear with each other and forgive one
another if any of you has a grievance against
someone. Forgive as the Lord forgave you.

COLOSSIANS 3:13

Forgiveness doesn't mean that we forget a wrong someone did to us, nor does it make us okay with it. It simply allows us to experience more emotional freedom as we move on with our lives without continued feelings of anger or desire for revenge.

Journal about a time someone forgave you and how it made you feel.

Opposition

Consider Him who endured such
opposition from sinners, so that
you will not grow weary and lose heart.

HEBREWS 12:3

When people oppose us, it can be helpful to remember that people also opposed Jesus and He can empathize with all the feelings we experience as a result.

What, if anything, changes for you as you dwell on this fact? How can you remember the opposition Jesus faced to change your response to opposition from others in your own life?

....

....

....

....

....

Conflict

All who rage against you will surely
be ashamed and disgraced; those who
oppose you will be as nothing and perish.
Though you search for your enemies,
you will not find them. Those who wage war
against you will be as nothing at all.

ISAIAH 41:11-12

God reminds us that in this world we will have trouble; to counter
this, He also comforts us with His promise of protection. It's
impossible to please everyone all the time, but God only asks us to
please *Him*.

How can mindfulness of God's power and sovereignty help you
avoid stress and anxiety when conflict with others arises?

....

....

Projecting

But instead, one brother takes another
to court—and this in front of unbelievers!
The very fact that you have lawsuits
among you means you have been completely
defeated already. Why not rather be wronged?
Why not rather be cheated? Instead,
you yourselves cheat and do wrong,
and you do this to your brothers and sisters.

1 CORINTHIANS 6:6–8

Oftentimes the things that bother us most about other people are things that we also struggle with. God wants us to examine ourselves and deal first with our own shortcomings.

Journal about what has been bothering you about others lately, and see if you can find any evidence of those struggles in your life.

Helping Others

Do not withhold good from those
to whom it is due, when it is in your power
to act. Do not say to your neighbor,
"Come back tomorrow and I'll give it
to you"—when you already have it with you.

PROVERBS 3:27–28

God created us to be dependent on Him, but it also pleases Him when we show up to help others.

Who in your life is struggling right now, and what is making life challenging for them? List some ways you can help and encourage them. Choose one and put it into practice today.

Defensiveness

Who will bring any charge against those
whom God has chosen? It is God who justifies.
Who then is the one who condemns?
No one. Christ Jesus who died—more than
that who was raised to life—is at the right
hand of God and is also interceding for us.

ROMANS 8:33-34

When someone accuses you of something, can you resist the urge to rush to defend yourself? Instead, can you pause for a moment and remind yourself that you have nothing to prove?

Journal about a time when you felt you needed to defend yourself. How might things have gone better if you had simply trusted God to intercede for you?

Practice: Beginning to Set Boundaries

If there are certain people, places, and things that have made it difficult for us to set boundaries in the past, we can change this, but first we have to acknowledge our part in the relationship dynamic. Though we may not be able to control other people, we can always control ourselves and our reactions.

With that in mind, write down some ways you have allowed people to take advantage of you or mistreat you in the past. What are the ways in which you have previously not stood up for yourself? List some reasons you might have allowed people to treat you that way.

If you have resentment toward a person or situation, it's time to set a boundary. Decide what you need, and practice asking for it before dealing directly with the person in question. Role-play the conversation with a person you trust or a therapist to help you feel more comfortable. Then, once you have expressed your boundary, plan a natural consequence should the person choose to violate your boundary, and commit to following through.

Closing Prayer

Heavenly Father, I am grateful that You created me to be in relationship with other people. Please bless my family relationships and my friendships. I thank You for all the amazing people in my life who love and care for me. You have greatly blessed me by putting them in my life. Please help me see ways that I can reflect Your love back to them each day.

Make me someone who diligently pursues peace with all people. Please help me navigate my relationships with grace when they become difficult. Help me slow down and seek You first before I respond in a way that might hurt someone.

Give me guidance on how to make my relationships stronger and on what I can do to love others even better than I do now. Help me lean on You for wisdom when I have disagreements with people or when any relational troubles arise. I pray that You will help me show Your love to people in a way that glorifies You. Let me be someone who exudes kindness and patience, even with difficult people. Help me receive Your grace when I fall short in any of these areas.

In Jesus's name, amen.

Resources

BOOKS

13 Things Mentally Strong People Don't Do by Amy Morin, LCSW
This book covers 13 ways of thinking that can be problematic
for our mental health, as well as practical ways to overcome them.

31 Days to Managing Your Moods by Cathleen Bearse, LCSW
This book will inspire and encourage you to make the positive
changes necessary to experience present-moment peace and
joy over the course of one month.

52-Week Mental Health Journal by Cynthia Catchings, LCSW-S,
LCSW-C, MSSW
This guided journal gives you 52 weeks of prompts and
self-reflection focused on reducing stress, increasing connection to others, and finding meaning and purpose in your life.

Choose Joy by Kay Warren
Sometimes it can be difficult to feel happy when we encounter difficult life circumstances; God invites us to instead
choose joy.

The Mindful Day by Laurie J. Cameron
Learn how to incorporate mindfulness into each and every
part of your day with this helpful and practical guide.

ONLINE

National Alliance on Mental Illness
NAMI.org
This website shares mental health resources and can connect
you with support groups in your area.

Psychology Today
PsychologyToday.com
This website offers helpful information and articles, and it can
help you find a licensed therapist near you.

Scripture Index

Acknowledgments

I'm so grateful for all the people who cheered me on while creating this journal, especially my incredibly supportive husband, Matthew.

Thank you to Joshua, Samuel, Jayden, and baby K. Mama loves you so very much.

To my editor, Eun H. Jeong, and everyone at Rockridge Press: I appreciate you.

And above all, thanks be to God.

About the Author

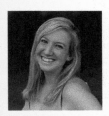 CATHLEEN BEARSE, LCSW, is a psychotherapist, online course creator, and blogger. She hosts the *Fearless Fostering* podcast, where she provides weekly education and encouragement for foster and adoptive moms. She lives in Connecticut with her husband and four children. You can find Cathleen on Instagram @fearless_fostering or on her website, FearlessFostering.com.